Watch with Me

Inspiration for
a life in hospice care

Watch with Me

*Inspiration for
a life in hospice care*

Cicely Saunders

Mortal Press

Acknowledgements

'Watch with Me' first appeared in *Nursing Times*, vol. 61, no. 48 (November 1965), pp. 1615–17, copyright EMAP Healthcare, 1965, and is reproduced by permission of *Nursing Times*; 'Faith' was first published in *The Guildford Lectures 1974* (Guildford Cathedral, 1974), pp. 1–7, and appears here by kind permission of the Dean and Chapter, Guildford Cathedral; 'Facing Death' was first published in *The Way*, October 1984, pp. 296–304, and appears here by kind permission of the publisher; 'A Personal Therapeutic Journey', from a series of articles entitled 'Into the valley of the shadow of death', first appeared in the *British Medical Journal*, vol. 313 (21–28 December 1996), pp. 1599–1601, and appears here by kind permission of the BMJ Publishing Group; 'Fresh Springs' by Sr Gillian Mary S.S.C. (Society of the Sacred Cross) from *Beyond the horizon*, edited by Dame Cicely Saunders (Darton, Longman & Todd, 1990), p. 79, appears here by kind permission of the author.

First published in 2003 by
MORTAL PRESS
PO Box 625, Sheffield, S1 3GY, UK

info@mortalpress.com
www.mortalpress.com

British Library Cataloguing-in-Publication Data
A British Library CIP Record is available.

ISBN 0-9544192-2-7
Typeset in Bembo by BBR Solutions Ltd, Chesterfield.
Printed on acid-free paper in the UK by the Alden Group Ltd, Oxford.

Buy this and other Mortal Press titles from www.mortalpress.com.

Contents

vii   Foreword *by David Clark*

1   Watch with Me

9   Faith

19   Facing Death

31   A Personal Therapeutic Journey

39   Consider Him

Foreword
by David Clark

The name of Cicely Saunders is synonymous with the creation of the modern hospice movement. Hospice care is one of the great social innovations of the twentieth century and most of her adult years have been dedicated to its development. Probably the first physician anywhere to devote an entire professional career to the care of dying people, her work has stimulated new services throughout the world and she is a long-standing advocate of the importance of research and teaching. Underpinning the entire scheme however, have been some significant religious and spiritual concerns that she brings to her practice and her writing. These have evolved and deepened over time and have been shaped by the prevailing theological and philosophical landscape, to which she continues to be open as a source of ideas. This book takes us into these concerns and helps us to understand not only how she came into this work, but how she has sustained her involvement over the decades. It provides a unique insight into the inspiration for a life in hospice care.

Cicely Saunders was born on 22 June 1918 and at the age of 20 went to read politics, philosophy and economics at Oxford University. In 1940 she interrupted academic studies to become a student nurse at the Nightingale Training School at London's St Thomas's Hospital. When a back injury forced her to leave nursing, she returned to Oxford and qualified in 1944 with a wartime BA and a Diploma in Public and Social Administration. She then commenced training as a hospital almoner, or medical social worker.

It was in this role in a large London hospital that she cared for David Tasma, a refugee from Poland and a survivor of the Warsaw ghetto. Within the short time that they knew each other he proved an inspiration to Cicely Saunders, so much so, that their professional relationship turned into a deep friendship. When he died, on 25 February 1948, David Tasma left Cicely Saunders with a gift of £500 and the encouragement, 'I'll be a window in your Home'—a reference to their discussions about the possibility of alternative places in which to care for those close to the end of life.

She determined immediately to learn more about the needs of those with a terminal illness and began work as a volunteer in St Luke's, a home for the dying in Bayswater, London. There followed the momentous decision to study medicine, starting in 1951 and qualifying in her late thirties. In 1958 she took up a position as Research Fellow at St Mary's School of Medicine, conducting work at St Joseph's Hospice in Hackney, in the East End of London. Here she laid down the basic principles of modern hospice care, developing a systematic approach to pain control in terminally ill patients; giving attention to their social, emotional and spiritual needs; and teaching what she knew to other people.

Soon she made plans to build her own modern hospice: one that would focus on three linked activities—clinical care, teaching and research. She gathered around her a group of supporters who helped to work out her ideas in detail, and she travelled to the United States and other countries to promote and refine her thinking. There were huge barriers to be overcome, yet after eight years of fund-raising, planning and promotion, St Christopher's Hospice was opened to its first patients in 1967. As she often remarked afterwards, 'it took me 19 years to build the Home round the window'.

For the next 18 years Cicely Saunders was the medical director of the hospice she had created. She quickly expanded its services to include home care; she promoted research into pain control and into the efficacy of the programme; she developed a centre for specialist education; and she was the author of a steady stream of publications. The work was acclaimed internationally and she was awarded many prizes and honours from numerous countries. St Christopher's received thousands of visitors each year and became a beacon of inspiration for others who came there to study, to develop clinical skills and to conduct research in the burgeoning field that had now come to be known as palliative care.

In 1985 Cicely Saunders retired from full-time work at the hospice, yet remained active in her writing, teaching and support for developments in palliative care. Her eightieth birthday was celebrated in 1998 with a conference in her honour at the Royal College of Physicians, London. In the year 2000 she stood down from the position of Chairman at St Christopher's to take on the role of President/Founder and to give time to assist in the development of a major new initiative, the Cicely Saunders Foundation.

In July 2003, just after her eighty-fifth birthday, Cicely Saunders spoke to a packed gathering in London's Westminster Cathedral Hall. The lecture was part of a series concerned with the spiritual exercises of St Ignatius and their relationship to various forms of human experience and daily living. She drew upon her own spiritual journey, from a search for God through wartime nursing, to her work as the founder and leader of the world's first modern hospice, all couched within her mature reflections on spiritual understanding in later life.

Soon afterwards, Dame Cicely asked me if I thought the lecture might be published. On reading it I certainly felt that it should find a wider audience. At the same time the piece awakened in me echoes of her earlier writings, and I found myself hunting back to locate these important antecedents to this most recent offering. The effect was uplifting and I was soon able to trace a particular and deeply enduring preoccupation: running through several published works was a concern for the relationship between personal biography, the spiritual life and an ethics of care. In each instance this was narrated in the first person, drew upon a range of religious and philosophical influences, and was underpinned throughout with a primary motivation: the care of specific individuals in the face of imminent death. In short, these were writings of the deepest importance within the contemporary hospice and palliative care canon.

So it became clear that the publication of the 2003 lecture would be richly enhanced by locating it in a pre-existing framework of related material. In discussion with Dame Cicely, a selection of five works was chosen—as it turned out, beginning in 1965, and with one piece from each subsequent decade. And so it was that this engaging book came about.

The opening chapter here is taken from a talk given to the 1965 Annual General Meeting of St Christopher's Hospice and was published just before Advent. It begins with reference to the foundations of St Christopher's, laid earlier that year. Seen more widely, these foundations have varied forms: the interest and money contributed; the people involved; the work previously done in the care of dying people. The most important foundation stone however is found in words spoken in the garden of Gethsemane: 'Watch with me'. The article can therefore be seen as a preparation for what will be encountered in the hospice: patients who don't want to die; mental suffering; the need for a sense of community and religious foundation. 'Watch with me' sums up the demands that lay ahead in 1965, but also echoes throughout the pages of this book, a recurring theme in each of the pieces.

In a 1974 lecture at Guildford Cathedral, Cicely Saunders was asked to speak on the subject of faith. The difficulty of the assignment is acknowledged, but so too is a source of inspiration: the patients from whom she has learned so much and for whom she tries to speak. David Tasma's request for 'what is in your mind and in your heart' created an obligation to do something about the care of the dying, however long it might take. This is linked to the idea of faith as obedience to a command; so that 'It is in action that faith is seen, grows and develops'. The creation of St Christopher's, 19 years after David Tasma's death and when his donation of £500 had been extended to £500,000, is one such example. At the same time it is also important to beware the faith that may simply become foolhardiness. In an interestingly topical reference for the period, Tolkien's metaphors of the quest are taken up here to illustrate how, despite the worst adversities, 'release comes unexpectedly and in the end all are seen to have played a part'. Yet faith can also be about letting go, or about receiving with open hands, as well as being the giver.

Written for a Catholic journal in the mid-1980s, 'Facing Death' is a reflective piece containing the distillation of decades of personal experience in caring for the dying, coupled with some of the spiritual and intellectual influences that have been brought to bear on this work along the way. It deals with sudden and violent death, as well as death from cancer and other diseases. It shows how the dying person is embedded within a web of personal and family relationships, responsibilities and obligations and how these are influenced by culture and history. In particular it focuses on aspects of coming to terms with death, with or without some kind of faith, so that 'To face death is to face life and to come to terms with one is to learn much about the other'.

'A Personal Therapeutic Journey' appeared in the Christmas edition of the *British Medical Journal* in 1996. It has often been quoted since and must have been enjoyed by many readers. We are taken back to those busy wards at St Thomas's in wartime, with their demanding routines and limited armamentarium. Reflections on the use of the 'Brompton Cocktail' recall an era before the modern techniques of pain control. The subsequent role of hospices in advancing new understandings is highlighted and there is a reminder about Cicely Saunders's concept of 'total pain'—still surely the most important and original concept to emerge in the field of palliative care.

The collection is concluded wonderfully with 'Consider Him', the lecture of summer 2003. Again she returns to the themes of personal faith, the inspiration for therapeutic work, the lessons taught by individual patients and the need for community and fellowship in the care of dying people. Those already familiar with the achievements of Cicely Saunders will find in this piece and all of those that precede it here a splendid affirmation of her life and philosophy; they will also gain new insights into the evolution of her thinking and its relevance to contemporary debates in palliative care. Those less aware of her work will gain insights into a remarkable life, her abiding curiosity, and enduring energy. As a result they will come to understand a personal philosophy that has contributed so much to the landscape of modern care for dying people and their families.

These five pieces are much more than a set of personal reflections. They pose an enduring challenge to prevailing orthodoxies in the now established field of palliative care; they highlight what it means to care *about* as well as to care *for* patients; they raise questions about the nature of vocation and how it might be maintained across a professional lifetime; they speak to us across the decades about what it means to search for better ways of caring for the dying and how this can be achieved; and on every page they offer some observation or insight that is of continuing relevance to the philosophy and practice of contemporary end of life care.

In conversation with Dame Cicely in 2002, she talked at length about the four decades encompassed by the pieces in this book, and her evolving spiritual path over those years. 'In general,' she remarked, 'I don't believe so many things today as I did before; but my beliefs now are certainly held more deeply.' Whether or not one shares those beliefs, this is a book that should be read by anyone concerned about the care of dying people in the modern world.

'Watch with Me'

We can think about the foundations of St Christopher's in various ways. We can say that they consist of all the interest and the money that has been given and promised and that have made the building and the laying of the foundation stone possible. We can think about them as all the work that has ever been done in this field in the past by people other than ourselves and on which we will build our own work. We can think about them as the people who have gradually joined in thinking, praying and working for St Christopher's ever since the vision was first given more than 17 years ago. I think that you all know that I like best of all to think of St Christopher's as being founded on patients, those we have known and who are now safely through this part of their lives. One used to speak for all of them each time I told her of some meeting, as she said 'I'll be there'. Now I want to look at our foundations by taking one particular phrase which I believe expresses our ideals concerning St Christopher's.

Ideals and aims of St Christopher's

I am sure the most important foundation stone we could have comes from the summing up of all the needs of the dying which was made for us in the Garden of Gethsemane in the simple words 'Watch with me'. I think the one word 'watch' says

Taken from a talk given to the annual general meeting of St Christopher's Hospice, published in *Nursing Times*, vol. 61, no. 48 (November 1965), pp. 1615–17, copyright EMAP Healthcare, 1965, and reproduced by permission of *Nursing Times*.

many things on many different levels, all of importance to us. In the first place it demands that all the work at St Christopher's should stem from respect for the patient and very close attention to his distress. It means really looking at him, learning what this kind of pain is like, what these symptoms are like, and from this knowledge finding out how best to relieve them. It means continually gaining new skills, developing those already learnt from St Luke's Hospital and the writings of its founder Dr Howard Barrett, from all the work of St Joseph's Hospice and from discussion with many other people both here and in the USA. I have not found any individual place concentrating on these problems alone but many have helped to shed light on different facets of them and all this we want to bring together and develop into new skills in an area that is very greatly neglected.

'Not only skill but compassion also'

We want to plan and carry out research in the relief of distress such as has not been done anywhere else, so far as I have been able to discover. It is often easier in a specialist setting to go on learning in this way and by building what we think is an ideal unit we hope to be able to help not only our own patients but to raise standards generally and also to stimulate others to think about these problems. A patient comes to my mind here, a young woman who said, 'You seem to understand the pain from *both* sides.' Our aim in learning such understanding is to give the kind of relief described by another woman who said, 'It was *all* pain but now it's gone and I am free.'

Seventeen years ago a young Pole died and left me £500 to be 'a window in your Home'. This was the very beginning of St Christopher's. I also remember his saying, 'I only want what is in your mind and in your heart.' This was echoed years later by another Pole who said to us, 'Thank you. And not just for your pills but for your heart.' I think both of them showed that they wanted not only skill but compassion also. They needed warmth and friendship as well as good technical care. I think our understanding of what real watching means must include this.

We have, indeed, to learn what this pain is like. Still more we have to learn what it feels like to be so ill, to be leaving life and its activity, to know that your faculties are failing, that you are parting from loves and responsibilities. We have to learn how to feel 'with' patients without feeling 'like' them if we are to give the kind of listening and steady support that they need to find their own way through.

Here again comes a key phrase I have often quoted, 'I look for someone to look as if they are trying to understand me.' These patients are not looking for pity and indulgence but that we should look at them with respect and an expectation of courage, a heritage from seeing people like the woman who said to me, 'You can tell them all that it was *all right*.' She was not going though a strange, dramatic or just unlucky experience, to be written up as such with sentimentality or sensationalism, but an all-too-common experience such as ordinary people have always faced and somehow managed to come through.

'I do not *want* to die'

We will be seeing patients who go along the path which leads from the honest but wistful plea, 'I do not *want* to die, I do not *want* to die', to the quiet acceptance of 'I only want what is right'. We will not only see acceptance but also a very real joy, the true gaiety of someone who has gone through doubt, fear and unwillingness and come out the other side. I remember coming away from the bedside of a man who had come along that difficult path just about an hour before he died and saying to myself—'He looked *amused*'—and he really did. Certainly we are going to see hard things, but we are also going to see rewards and compensations and insight given to our patients here and now and we will see an extraordinary amount of real happiness and even light-heartedness.

Planning an ideal unit is not enough to interpret all the meaning of the word 'watch' if teaching is not a vital part of what we do. We want St Christopher's to be a place where all kinds of people can join us to learn from our experience and learn from our patients with us. This does not mean burdening the patients with the demands of continual bedside teaching. It does mean that you can give them an interest I know they enjoy if it is done in the right way. It can also reveal a new purpose in what is happening to them and what they are doing themselves. Certainly they are not all going to be saints. Some will be, indeed, and we will be very honoured and helped by their coming to us. Others will be splendidly maddening and I have no time to suggest the various crises with which we are going to have to cope. But who is to say who does the best—the person whose last weeks are the crown of a life of devotion, the young girl who makes the whole ward into a party for months on end and never shows you how much it costs her, or the old man who just manages to stop grumbling for his last 10 days or so? Certainly we will never fail to learn from them and some of the things that we will learn may surprise our future staff. Work here will not just be solemn. Rather I would just say it will be real and reality is gay and funny as well as serious. Above all, it will never be dull.

Being there

'Watch with me' means, still more than all our learning of skills, our attempts to understand mental suffering and loneliness and to pass on what we have learnt. It means also a great deal that cannot be understood. Those words did not mean 'understand what is happening' when they were first spoken. Still less did they mean 'explain' or 'take away'. However much we can ease distress, however much we can help the patients to find a new meaning in what is happening, there will always be the place where we will have to stop and know that we are really helpless. It would be very wrong indeed if, at that point, we tried to forget that this was so and to pass by. It would be wrong if we tried to cover it up, to deny it and to delude ourselves that we were always successful. Even when we feel that we can do absolutely nothing, we will still have to be prepared to stay.

'Watch with me' means, above all, just 'be there'. I remember the patient who said of the people who had really helped her, 'They never let you down. They just keep on coming.' I also remember she described the way God had met her by saying, 'He sends me people.' I am quite certain that St Christopher's has to learn to be a place where people do not let you down but instead give the feeling of reassurance and safety that comes from faithfulness.

I think from this need especially stems the demand that we should grow into a real community. It is very important that we should be a group of people who have confidence in each other and that St Christopher's should be the kind of family and home that can give the welcome and hospitality of a good home, where people are accepted as themselves and can relax in security. It must also be a place where everyone knows that the individual contributions matter and that there is no hierarchy of importance in what is done. Who will know what or who matters most to an individual patient as his manifold problems are dealt with by various members of such a group? There is a kind of compassionate matter-of-factness that develops in such a place and in this the hard-pressed worker is not overwhelmed by her own responsibilities.

The community of all men

Above all, I think that it is here that we see the very great need for a religious foundation. We must remember that we belong to the much wider community of the whole Church, to the whole communion of saints and, indeed, to the whole community of all men. It is because of this that St Christopher's is ecumenical and undenominational. We will welcome people of all sorts and kinds and be of all sorts and kinds ourselves. We are not emphasising that there is just one way but rather that there is one Person coming in many ways.

The same words 'Watch with me' remind us also that we have not begun to see their meaning until we have some awareness of Christ's presence both in the patient and in the watcher. We will remember his oneness with all sufferers, for that is true for all time whether they recognise it here or not. As we watch them we know that he has been here, that he still is here and that his presence is redemptive.

Reinterpreting an old truth

We do not help patients through this part of life by denying that it can sometimes be very hard. We do not see it truly if we just think somewhat vaguely of immortality and 'going on' rather than of death followed by resurrection. Dying followed by rebirth has been a dominant theme of man's religion from the very beginnings of belief. For Christians this has once and for all been summed up and made truth in Christ himself. I believe that it is very important that this message should be shown at St Christopher's in every possible way for it has hardly any meaning to a great majority of people in Great Britain today. This stands out with sad vividness in Geoffrey Gorer's survey, *Death, grief and mourning in contemporary Britain*. It is a truth which needs to be reinterpreted in terms that are relevant to all those who will come to us, to the patients, to their relations and to all the visitors. Perhaps we may have a contribution to make to the 'new theology' as we learn about this very simply, seeing this truth, this Person, meeting people today.

Through symbols and sacraments

Christ will be present in all the skills that we learn and in symbols and sacraments of all kinds. These will include the sacraments of the cup of cold water and the washing of the disciples' feet. All these things will speak silently to the patients about God's love for them. So too will the whole planning and decoration of the building itself, thought out over a very long period with our architect and carried out by him with great insight and imagination. Especially, I think it will be shown in the planning of the chapel and in all the pictures, the symbols and the sculpture that are being created specially for us by artists who share this faith with us. It is very important that this message should be shown in these different ways. I have seen again and again how receptive patients are to the things they look at when they are not able to bear with talking any longer. Often it is important that very little should be said at all because it is so easy to interrupt a real message.

So much of our communication with people is done

without words but I think this is especially so with the very ill. The patient who says soon after her admission, 'It is marvellous to begin to feel safe again', has been met by the atmosphere and by the things she lies and looks at just as much as by the nursing and by the drugs and relief she is given. In a whole climate of safety she finds her own key and her own meeting. We will see patients able to listen, perhaps for the first time, to something that has been said to them all their lives but for which they have somehow never had time for real attention.

I have been impressed again and again at St Joseph's by the way patients will lie and look at a picture or a crucifix and how much these can then say to them. I believe that it is very important that these should be works created now, by artists who are interpreting these truths in the context of the world today. I am especially glad that this growing emphasis on art for St Christopher's has given us connections with Poland once again, a link that has been there from the beginning and forged again and again.

'My bags are packed …'

I think all of us remember the words of Pope John when he said, 'My bags are packed and I can leave with a tranquil heart at any moment.' I think that this is how we pray for all the patients who come to us. We remember that some of them are already ill, frail, lonely or despairing and pray for them now. Others are busy and have no thought of calamity. Perhaps only in calamity are they going to find the meaning of the whole of the rest of their lives. I think that we should pray that we will be able to make it possible for them to pack their bags with the right things, pack them with what matters, with what *they* need; that while they are here they will find all that they should of reconciliation, fulfilment and meaning as they go through this last part of their lives.

… to be silent, to listen, to be there

I have tried to sum up the demands of this work we are planning in the words 'Watch with me'. Our most important foundation for St Christopher's is the hope that in watching we should learn not only how to free patients from pain and distress, how to understand them and never let them down, but also how to be silent, how to listen and how just to be there. As we learn this we will also learn that the real work is not ours at all. We are building for so much more than ourselves. I think if we try to remember this we will see that the work is truly to the greater glory of God.

Faith

One of the first rules for taking examinations is to 'read the question'. What does it mean? Why is it asked and what is the examiner trying to find out? In preparing myself for the first of your lectures for this autumn I found myself doing a similar exercise. Why was I asked to do this? What is expected of me? Fortunately Canon Telfer was specific and has given me valuable help in trying to tackle a daunting assignment.

I am not expected to talk of faith as a theologian. Indeed the main reason for my being here at all is the fact that I am not a theologian. I was invited as a member of the laity, as one of the nonprofessionals. Above all, I am invited to represent St Christopher's Hospice, with the background of its hopes, its beginnings and its day-to-day working among the long-term sick and dying people. Our work has been seen as showing something of the nature of faith, and what our patients have been teaching us as having much to say to ordinary living.

I have been here before, and perhaps some of you may remember Louie, who had been in bed all her life, with fragile bones. One day, when she knew that she was dying and we were talking about it, I said to her, 'What's the first thing you'll say to Him, Louie?' and she said, without hesitation, 'I know You.' She *knew* Him, she did not just know *about* Him. For her, faith was loving trust rather than belief in doctrine or concepts, in fact it was hardly in words at all. It is from this kind of faith that I want

First published in *The Guildford Lectures 1974* (Guildford Cathedral, 1974), pp. 1–7, and appears here by kind permission of the Dean and Chapter, Guildford Cathedral.

to begin, for Louie is one of the many people, nearly all of them patients, through whom the vision of St Christopher's was given and in whom much of its life continues. I would not have dared to accept this assignment if I had not felt I could, and should, try to speak for them.

When our own knowing Him seems so pathetically overwhelmed by lesser concerns, again and again we find inspiration in coming back to our patients. About two weeks ago you may have seen David Frost interviewing four of them, each talking of faith in different ways and allowing the Infinite God to shine through a finite person, through what was becoming an increasingly fragile existence. Since that programme was made Mr Vincent has been losing further movement in his hands and Mary has gone quietly, without pain, into Paradise.

St Christopher's began when David Tasma, a lonely Polish man from the Warsaw ghetto, talked of his needs with me when I was still a social worker. When he left £500 'to be a window in your Home', and when he said, 'I only want what is in your mind and in your heart', he talked of his hopes for people who would come after him, and of certainties he would not see. Through him a demand was made on me—I had to go and do something about it, however long it might take.

It was 19 years before the first patient came past David Tasma's window and the first members of staff began to try to give what was in their minds and in their hearts, to bring all they could summon of skill and friendship to relieve the manifold distress that has ever since been coming into St Christopher's. For me, his words put together two of the many descriptions of faith which I could have taken for my texts. In the first, Jesus is told by the centurion that He need only say the word for his servant to be healed and the centurion is ready to go back home and find it so. Jesus looked at him and said, 'I have not found so great a faith'. In the second, the writer to the Hebrews defines faith, 'Faith gives substance to our hopes and makes us certain of realities we cannot see' (New English Bible). Or as Phillips translates it, 'Faith means putting our full confidence in the things we hope for, it means being certain of things we cannot see.'

The story of the centurion speaks of committing yourself to a person, of seeing in Him such compassionate authority that you are prepared to do anything He says; the second tells of going ahead with a conviction, putting your trust in it and going on into the action it impels. I think that these two 'faiths' are the same, certainly the action they imply is similar. This faith is obedience to a command, and surely nothing can command us quite so inexorably as an inner conviction. It is in action that faith is seen, grows and develops.

It is not at all straightforward. I remember once, when a most unwelcome piece of publicity was about to hit us, I went to see a very mature and supportive patient to ask for her prayers, afraid that we had really made a mistake in deciding to allow a film to be made in the Hospice. She said firmly, 'Never go back on guidance,' and sent me back to do all I could in talking to the reporters concerned. 'No man, having put his hand to the plough and looking back, is fit for the Kingdom of God ...' does not mean that faith cannot be mistaken in guidance but is a firm reminder as to which direction we should be looking if we are to get back on the way.

After a few years spent learning from patients in St Luke's, Bayswater and in becoming a doctor, I began work on the control of pain in St Joseph's Hospice. There I met Louie, Alice, Terry and others who, like David Tasma, became convinced that what they saw as a promise which would meet their own special needs could indeed become a concrete reality. The words, 'Now you've got to get on with it' were unmistakable. Later, potential staff began to appear and to bring their own contributions of faith and talents. Nineteen years after David's promise, the Home, St Christopher's Hospice, was built round the window—the £500 had become £500,000.

It was rather like a sermon I heard once in Westminster Abbey, for which I can't give due credit as I have forgotten who was the preacher. He described the faith that would move a mountain and cast it into the sea in what was for me a new way. One person, looking at a mountain above a cliff, became convinced that it should be moved into the sea. So he took a wheelbarrow and a spade and began, load by load, to push it over the cliff. For a while he kept on alone; then one or two others, instead of mocking him, thought that this was something that needed doing, and joined him. Later others saw it as a possibility and joined also. Eventually the mountain was no more.

Such action can be the simple obedience to God's command. But we have to be careful for we are great self-deceivers. Faith may be foolhardiness and Jesus has some firm things to say about counting the cost. It can also be a cloak in which we dress our own ambitions. We know ourselves so little and we know God still less. Sometimes the way of finding Him is by a readiness to plumb our own inner depths. If we can find our own wellspring of being we may have found something of our link with the maker of all things. But another, and for many of us a less hazardous way, is in knowing others. We are more likely to find our Incarnate God in others than in words or concepts. I believe that the response to His call through patients, in their need and their achievement, has been a place of safety for us. We are less likely to think of ourselves as 'just a stick for God to use' and so end up as no more than a stick to beat others—driving them to act to our satisfaction and not in answer to a call from our Father and theirs. The constant call for love is a more reliable guide for faith than some 'illuminations'.

Faith has been compared to belief in fairy tales. Those who make this comparison perhaps do not always know how truly they speak. We love the archetypal story of the journey which goes through innumerable dangers, finds unexpected helpers and then is suddenly set right in what Professor Tolkien calls the Eucatastrophe, the happy ending which upturns all the evil so apparently undefeatable and ends in the fruitfulness of living happily ever after. Abraham and Moses each set out on their journey, not knowing where or how they were going, and became fathers of us all. Surely the attraction of Tolkien's Ring trilogy is the complex and haunting journey of his fellowship. He will not have it that his story is an allegory but we may find in such tales what we will. Readers will remember the confusion of ambition and self-seeking that hinders some of the travellers and that it is

Frodo's simple obedience to a call he scarcely understands and Sam's single-hearted love for Frodo himself which leads the two of them to fulfil the quest on their own. The final dogged stage of their journey is heart-rending but heartening reading for any who see no sign of the happy ending for themselves—and a fine description of the simplicity of the faith which has nothing left to do but simply hang on … 'having done all, to stand'. Those who reach this place may find, like Frodo, that God's way of release comes unexpectedly and in the end all are seen to have played a part.

Faith is not only doing and not only keeping on, however doggedly. It is also letting go. Frodo and Sam come back, but Frodo has to give up to others the peace he has won for them. Faith comes to the place of taking hands off, of letting go. Sometimes this is in the desperation of the weariness of the friend who said to me last week, 'I'll do whatever my surgeon says, I've felt rotten for so long now, I leave the decision entirely to him.' Sometimes it is in being ready to receive instead of constantly being the giver. I spoke last time I was here of a certain Mr P who was in the Hospice for a few months and who came back to a trust in God during his stay. When I was giving him some photographs of himself taken at our Boxing Day party he wanted to pay me, I wanted to give them as a present. We both wanted to give, neither wanted to receive. I finally held out my hand to say, 'I suppose that is what life is about, learning to receive.' He put both his hands out next to mine, palms upwards, and said, 'That's what life is about, four hands held out together.' Clenched hands are lonely, unrelenting, closed in (even to the agony of Pincher Martin's clawed fists as they resist the dark lightning of God's love in William Golding's compelling novel). Open hands are vulnerable, accepting and a symbol of the faith that can receive and be blessed, over and above all our imagining. They are ready for freedom and for spontaneity. Jesus tells us that to enter His Kingdom we must become like children … surely in their trust and the openness that is so ready to grow in love. I think that is why the crime of taking away a child's trust has such a devastating condemnation from Him and why we respond to the interpretations of the psychologists as they tell us of the importance of those early years in the growth of a basic trust in life.

What of a child whose trust is betrayed or who is deprived from the beginning of his chance to open up to others, whose potential for love and spontaneity becomes twisted and bitter? What of all the questions of faith? 'Why should this happen to the one I love?' A harder and more common question than 'Why should this happen to me?' What too of all the seemingly random miseries of war, greed and materialism? All the wastes and sorrows of the world?

Those who are busy in trying to relieve suffering are fortunate because the question 'how?' overwhelms the 'why?' and for that first question there is an answer, demanding though it may well be on the questioner. It seems to me that it is the question asked by the Good Samaritan and the answers lead us into the sacraments of the cup of cold water and of taking a towel, sacraments which strengthen the faith of many who do not at this moment find the more liturgical sacraments helpful.

Faith grows also when people ask the question 'how?' at the approach of the passivities and diminishments of illness and of dependence of all kinds. I remember a man who said, 'I do not understand, I can do nothing for you, I can only hurt you,' and when, later, just as he was dying, he was told, 'Please believe me—it is you who has been giving to me,' he could say with simplicity, 'I believe you.' Love links the two kinds of faith, the faith of trust and the faith of belief. Love is the key to the answers of all the questions of 'why?' for in love we learn to wait for the full answers. That same man, when he knew that he was going to die, said one day, 'I do not *want* to die ...'. The sharing of the thought of Gethsemane seemed too far away to help at that moment, but when a few weeks later he said in another context, 'I only want what is right', he had not only come through, he had brought Gethsemane into today and Christ had triumphed there once more. We all have our cloud of witnesses around us if only we will be more ready to see them, and hold out our hands to receive what God has to give us through them.

Faith is a strange word: it needs to be linked to another; faith-and-obedience, faith-and-love are not easily disentangled. When Louie said, 'I know You', she said it in the humble trust of love. You can be ashamed, you can be wrong and admit it, with someone who truly loves you. For then there is no more need of self-protection, you can open your fists into hands, you can move from doing into being, and be yourself.

Being vulnerable in trustful love is the foundation of the obedience of faith and of the place where you can receive although you cannot give. It seems to me that it is a description of faith when the Psalmist says, 'What reward shall I give unto the Lord: for all the benefits that he hath done unto me? I will receive the cup of salvation: and call upon the name of the Lord' (Psalm 116:11, 12).

There is great strength in weakness accepted and perhaps it sums up much of what theology has to teach in a way more comprehensible than words. Mr Vincent showed his two precious oil paintings to David Frost on television and the camera caught the horse and cart going down the village street at Chilham. Then Mr Vincent held his hands out, showed the deformity of increasing paralysis and said, 'It's progressive …'. He also said, 'It's suffering that God sends. You just have to accept it.' He has the right to say this because he has come on a long journey and God has been with him all the way. It is not the infliction of punishment or a heartless trial imposed from a distance. It is God's bearing from within Mr Vincent of his disease. In his case we do not know of any cause and no cure as yet. There are some diseases which arise from our way of life, others from the surprisingly few aberrations of the incredible subtlety of the cells of our bodies. It may help us to answer our questions 'why?' if we remember these facts and can accept that chance and accident are part of the world we know and will hit apparently haphazardly. But we have not yet come very far. If we added, 'We do not know why God allows this, but we do know that He will share it; and that as He does so He will redeem and transform it', then we are beginning to join Mr Vincent. But he is ready, from his experience, to use the shorthand of saying that God sent the suffering of his paralysis. He says so without bitterness because in it he has found new depths of the faithfulness of God and sees the whole as coming from His hand.

But Mr Vincent has left us far behind. He is also a practising Christian and his faith has much of the explicitness of belief. This raises a new set of questions. Is it not enough to live with open hands and to care about the constant learning to trust so as to be able to start a new beginning after each failure of love? Is it not enough faith for today if we are truly more concerned to be the kind of person we are meant to be than to remain stuck in the kind of doing and grasping in which our lives are spent? And, even if we believe in God, can we not accept that all religions speak of Him? Why do we Christians point to 'the faith' and say that to know God means to know a peculiarly personal God who has done certain things in history?

Many among those who admit to a love and longing for God in their hearts stop short of the claims and demands of such an outrageous particularity. How in all the immensity of space and time, in the complexities of our inheritance in evolution, and not least in all our misunderstandings of ourselves and our motives, can we possibly be expected to put our trust in such a 'once and for all'?

But perhaps here there is a likeness to the world we know, the home from which we start. Some of you may have watched the *Philpott File* from Guy's Hospital and seen how the years of training are summed up in one moment—as the surgeon puts the stitch into the valve in the open heart operation and as the sister takes the drain from the pericardium afterwards. We have seen how the whole of a lifetime of love is brought into one moment of meeting or farewell. Many of us have had a fleeting experience of the still wholeness of some kind of Eternal Now— in love or vision. The world of nature is full of moments like that recently described to me by a friend when a sudden panorama of mountains in the snow was seen in a flash alongside a few snowflakes on a dark ski glove. We know how everything centres down into a point. We live with the paradox of immensity and focus, both holding the truth. Cannot the Beyond in the Midst, the Prime Mover, the Ultimate Meaning, God Himself, come to such a point, the point of uttermost love? The greater the immensity, the finer, the more intense will be the focus.

There is no safe trust for us in the impassible, the unmoved, who sends help from above, we can only commit ourselves to the one who comes into the midst. And He who has the still wholeness within Him will absorb the long cry of a world's agony and so redeem it. The crucifixions which show nothing but agony and those which only illustrate quiet triumph are both true—but the darkness does not overcome finally. Sometimes we see glimpses of how this may be. I remember a few moments with someone much loved who was dying and how a visiting friend said, 'They look so awful when they are so ill, don't they.' But I did not see that at all—I saw only someone so nearly transparent to the God whom he loved and trusted. But that was a gift of love.

And finally, I suppose, that is what faith is, a gift of love, from love, to love. It is all much more simple than we think, though it is not easy. In fact, all I could ever say about faith as trust is so faint and far off I would have nothing to bring to you at all if I were not speaking of the gifts of David and Antoni and Mr Vincent and all the great multitude who came with their wheelbarrows to the mountain of getting St Christopher's built and working. This is not a place for assertions—only for an attempt to point to 'the drawing of this love and the voice of this Calling' that has slowly crystallised from a series of personal encounters.

At the Annunciation, Mary said, 'Let it happen as you say', and Christ came. I think that this is the word of faith, the 'I *know* you—I trust you', and the symbol of faith is the gesture of the hands open to receive. I cannot stop there; that is not the beginning. We love because He first loved us, because His hands are open to us. And they have in them for ever the prints of the nails.

Facing Death

You know, doctor, I never really thought that I was going to
die, I suppose we none of us do. But there does come a time
when you are ready to lay it down.

Lily, a patient in a hospice

We may face death intellectually, plan for insurance and
other practical matters, meditate on the death and
resurrection of Jesus and know well the Christian teachings. We
may (especially if we live in the USA), attend classes in 'Death
and dying', but all this is likely to fall short of a true facing of its
reality for ourselves. Even a ready facing of the little 'deaths' that
we meet in life is different in quality from its ending. Like Lily,
who had been disabled all her life, we do not really imagine that
we will die.

A true facing of death is not done once for all, it is an
individual journey for each person, a journey between those two
statements. However, though each one is unique, it takes place
across a broadly similar map. This journey is seen many times
over by those who work in hospice teams and from time to time
by all those in the caring professions. It implies work, often hard
work, on the part of all involved—the patient, his family and
friends and all the staff who are trying to help them. There may
be many problems to face but there are also achievements to be
made before the final letting go.

The modern voluntary euthanasia movement, now
established in different forms around the world, aims to make

---

First published in *The Way*, October 1984, pp. 296–304, and appears here by
kind permission of the publisher.

a legalised shortening of this time available to all who choose. While understanding such a desire when good care is not available and other priorities make it seem a distant dream, there are fundamental objections to this solution. The existence of a legal option for a quick way into death implies that there is little value any longer in the person who is dying and in the journey that he is making. Those who work close to people in this situation would affirm how much the dying person and his family would lose if time were to be cut short. Psychiatrists report that suicide is the most devastating of bereavements, leaving intolerable feelings of rejection and guilt for those left behind. But those who believe a legal right to end life would undermine the peace of mind and freedom from fear of many vulnerable people ('I am no better than a burden, I should not expect people to look after me'), have a responsibility to help people who are in such need. They may do this by active care, by neighbourly and social concern or by trying to encourage others to find how much may be gained by living until death comes. The 'sanctity of life' lies in each unique person.

Many deaths are sudden and give no opportunity for facing and coming to terms with what is happening. Such an unprepared entry into another world, and a judgment to face there, has been greatly feared in the past. Many people today seem to have lost this concern and give little thought to the idea of living each day in readiness. A lack of belief in anything beyond this world is now common, even though hospice workers frequently meet among families and friends a tentative hope that death is not the end of a loved person. They may express a vague expectation of 'a better world' or feel like Wandor, who wrote, 'On reflection, I'm not sure I would be better off believing in God. But when my mother died, I found that I was glad that some people still do.'[1] But even where there is no belief in another life that demands some preparation, there is surely still a place for completing work in this one. Time is often needed for a final summing up of what a life has meant and for reconciliations and meetings that can make a major difference to the family's journey through bereavement.

Violent deaths are sadly common, and shock and the absence of any time in which to begin to come to terms with loss make for difficult bereavements, especially when a child is killed by accident or even murder. The poignant contributions of the parents who share their experiences in the *Compassionate Friends Newsletter* show how much they need each other's understanding and help in a world where they are so frequently avoided and isolated by those around. And what of torture, disappearance, starvation and the many deprivations of a world so full of 'darkness and cruel habitations' (Psalm 74:20)? Suffering and death face us with much sorrow and many questions.

Death from cancer still seems to arouse a unique fear. Some consideration of its process and the ways of handling it that are seen in the hospices may be a helpful starting point from which to consider facing death more generally. Physical pain and other symptoms, decisions concerning appropriate aims of treatment, the frequently vexed question of whether to tell a patient the truth of his condition, the emotional responses of the family and even of some professionals to this particular diagnosis show many common problems in particularly sharp focus. Alongside the special threat of cancer we may consider the effects of some other progressive illness, the paralysis and loss of communication coupled with an alert mind of motor neurone disease and some strokes, the gradual loss of faculties of the organic dementias and of movement and independence in some rheumatic and similar painful disorders. In all these situations, the person concerned is facing a whole series of endings, of physical independence, of relationships, of hopes and future plans and of confidence in the meaning of his life. How can he be helped to endure them and to use the time that is left?

The progress of cancer is not as inexorable as some of the other diseases mentioned above. The development of treatments that may halt its progress or palliate its symptoms will lead the patient to 'hope against hope'. This may be tantalisingly unrealistic and merely bring the pain of hope deferred and it also poses the dilemma of when to cease fighting for life and accept the approach of death. Teilhard de Chardin presents this dilemma from a Christian point of view:

> We have come a long way, christianly speaking, from the justly criticised notion of 'submission to the will of God' which is in danger of weakening and softening the fine steel of the human will, brandished against all the powers of darkness and diminishment ... I can only unite myself to the will of God (as endured passively) when all my strength is spent ... Unless I do everything I can to advance or resist, I shall not find myself at the required point—I shall not submit to God as much as I might have done or as much as He wishes. If on the contrary, I persevere courageously, I shall rejoin God across evil, deeper down than evil; I shall draw close to Him.[2]

Many are afraid that the side effects of treatment will be worse than the disease itself, but yet feel guilty if they refuse it. Such decisions are never easy and patients do not always have the support they need in facing them. But once it has been decided that nothing more can be done to halt the progress of the disease there is a great deal that can be offered to ease its physical manifestations. The aim of pain control and the relief of other symptoms is that the patient should find his body and its needs less obtrusive, even when his activities are more and more curtailed by disease. Our bodies can have their essential integrity affirmed even in weakness and dependence and when careful attention is given to the analysis and treatment of its problems we can still feel that it is well regarded by others. A changing body image can be faced and accepted and a sense of personal worth be maintained even in the face of great physical loss.[3]

The successful control of terminal pain and other symptoms achieved during the past two decades, largely by the members of the hospice movement, has proved to be transferable to different settings, including the patient's own home. 'No patient should be allowed to die suffering, for pain can be relieved entirely in the majority and controlled satisfactorily in the rest.'[4] The public's preconceptions that all strong pain-killing drugs will lose their effect after inevitable increases in dose, and that at best patients will be sleepy and confused if pain is to be eased, have been shown to be untrue; and the teaching on how to use such drugs effectively is finally spreading widely into the general field.

The greatest sorrow of a dying patient is the ending of relationships and responsibilities. We live in our interchange with others and as encroaching weakness leads to the change of roles, as the wage earner can no longer work or the housewife has to hand all her activities in caring for the family to others, it is hard not to feel useless and humiliated. The family often takes readily the opportunity to repay debts of love and care but it is not easy to be perpetually at the receiving end of other people's concern and this must be given with sensitivity. This time can be used to heal bitterness and find reconciliation and, as at any time of crisis, this may take place at surprising speed. ('We lived a lifetime in three weeks.') But in order to do this well at least some of the truth of the situation has to be shared. Families often feel they must protect the dying person, but this is almost always misguided. The patient comes to know by other means and is then left even more isolated, unable to share his concern for others as well as for himself. To dissemble continually is inhibiting and exhausting for both sides.

However hard it may be to face the approaching parting it helps to stay with as much truth as possible to work through the anxiety and grief it brings. Some families have shared little during their life together, some people have spent their lives avoiding unpleasant realities and not every group will be successful. No one should be hurried through stark disclosures and we may have to wait while partial truths are gradually absorbed, but some shared awareness has again and again been seen to facilitate often surprising family growth.

Patients (and families) may continue to hope against hope, to take a 'day off' from truth by concentrating on a trip or a celebration, and still meet in depth at one and the same time. Nearly all of the many families who leave St Christopher's Hospice with new strengths after a patient's death are those who have been able to face their parting together. Bereavement will still be hard to come to terms with, but such memories will help to make this a creative process. The hospice team is ready to work singly or in groups with those who need special help for this long journey of sorrow.

To face death means to face the ending of hopes and plans. Pain is not only physical and social, it is also deeply emotional. Indeed, mental pain may be the most intractable of all. The anxiety over the disease and its treatments merges with the depression evoked by dwindling capacities. Most of us have reason to feel shame as we look back over our lives, but this is often confused and confounded with vague and irrational feelings of guilt among the very ill. Some people find themselves attacked by bouts of understandable anger or devastating despair. Yet clinical depression is comparatively rare among cancer patients and suicide uncommon.

Sadness is appropriate and should be faced and shared. It calls for a listener, rather than for drugs, although a combination of the two may help to lift an inhibiting load and enable a patient to tackle problems that had seemed unmanageable. When such treatment is carefully assessed and reviewed, this is not to manipulate the mind but to give it greater freedom and strength in facing reality. Sacraments announcing God's forgiveness may bring peace, or the acceptance of those around confirm this without words.

The greatest fear is of loss of control; yet even with an encroaching brain tumour or with failing mental powers the person may be helped to focus his attention and to respond in character to reality as he sees it. A daughter who described her father's slow disintegration of mind with loving yet scientific perception ended her moving description of his final achievement, 'Mind and body are inseparable, so far as we can tell, but experience suggests that they are no more than tools, and of much less account than the spirit whose purposes they serve.' The ending of that story was peaceful and once her father, in a remarkable moment of lucidity, had committed to others the welfare of the wife he loved 'he subsided afterwards into a quiet dementia which was like a rambling dream; vivid consciousness and depth of feeling were no longer present and I never felt another pang on his behalf.[5]

To face the increasing dementia of one much loved, often over years, is one of the hardest ways of facing their deaths. The carer, when the patient is at home, as so many are, or the relative who has handed care to often hurried and overworked professionals, faces a long, slow loss and frequently fails to receive needed support.

Anxiety, depression, anger and despair will also attack them and be exacerbated by exhaustion. The loss can gradually be accepted intellectually, emotionally and socially, and the agony of separation gradually lessened, but when death finally comes there will almost certainly still be much 'grief work' to do. Like the patient who is losing control and feels he is no longer his accustomed self, the bereaved have a new world to discover and accept. They cannot be hurried through the numbness, the emotional pain, the gradual realisation of the emptiness of loss and the final learning to live again. Some need much help in expressing their feelings all through this time and may finally need permission to stop grieving and allow other commitments to come around the gap.

Coming to terms with loss intensifies the ever present search for meaning.[6] The following extract from a diary dictated by Ramsey, who became blind and inhibited in speech from an inoperable brain tumour, shows how new vistas and even new faith can open up in the accepting surroundings of a hospice and how dying, like bereavement, can finally lead to new growth:

> 26.8.78: Amazingly enough, I believe I'm going to find a God. I don't know how it will happen precisely, but the sense that Jesus will find me and make me all that I am and more is not too far away, and the fact that He is coming at the time that I need Him most is amazing. To think that in such a short time and in my own way is coming to me Jesus Christ, that is, I hope, going to look after me, seems a most important thing, but I know it's going to be true. Annie is writing again, Jill is writing, people who know me love me and will stay with me forever, all will amaze me. Only now am I beginning to realise by thinking of God, what

He must know and think of how significant I am. I find it quite exciting to think of my future and to realise that Jesus is going to somehow make my life work and I wish I could have done it before, what does make me excited is the possibility of extending my life in this world or the next in all the ways that I now can.

Living of life and living of death was, I thought, to be a strange thing. I still think it's a strange thing. I want to try and make it a place where I am with everyone else when I am dead or alive, where it becomes a place that's not going to change. I don't know how it's going to happen, but I know it will happen. I don't know whether I'm going to die forever, but I know it doesn't really matter, because I'm going to be looked after, and everything that God wants me to do I will do to the best of my ability, and that is all that matters. I seem to be at the beginning of my life with God and that is amazing.[7]

Ramsey's syntax has gone but what he intended to say is clear. He died two weeks later, very peacefully.

We all need meaning in our lives, and to face death seems at first to face the loss of that meaning. Most people think of themselves in terms of what they do and find in that their place in the world. As their role is lost, as Ramsey lost his as a television producer, much of the integrity of the self seems to go too. Like many others, in his response to a totally new and extremely dependent situation, Ramsey found a new self. The body seems to have a wisdom of its own. If we follow its dictates, as its powers diminish so those of the spirit can find new strength and creativity. Those who search for a new and lasting truth in their lives find as Ramsey did that life can be laid down in hope, not of something indestructible in the self, but in trust in the God whose hands hold them in death as in life. For those who feel they can no longer pray from sheer weakness there is the holding by the prayer and love of others, 'where I am with everyone else' and above all, trust in the God who knows our ability. His judgment here and hereafter is a 'setting things right', and as we believe we will live on in the memories of those who love us so we can trust that our soul is safe to live on in the invincible love of God. And so we reach trust in the whole communion of saints, the household of God.

Ramsey was unusual in being able to express this in his late discovery of God. Many who have no words, or at least none of the traditional phrases, show by their attitude, their gestures and their response to those around them that they are reaching out trustfully to what they see as true. We believe that this reaching out brings them to 'The Truth'.

Paula, young, blonde and beautiful, had the cross removed from the niche in her room and put a horny little red devil in its place. She gave friendship and entertainment to us all for weeks but had apparently no time for spiritual questions. On her last night she asked a nurse what *she* believed. On being given a simple statement of faith in Christ, Paula said, 'I couldn't say I believed like that, not now, but would it be all right if I said that I hoped?' At that she took off the false eyelashes she wore night and day and gave them to the nurse to put away: 'I won't want these any more.'

But what of those who either do not have or do not take this opportunity? What of those who feel only the absence of God in their weakness or feel that they have lost their faith? Some can take Our Lord's words in the passion, the 'if it be possible' of Gethsemane and the 'why has Thou forsaken me?' from the cross and hold to them in darkness. Others who find no light in life will surely meet him in death:

> In His fourth word from the cross Christ went into the lowest depths to which man comes. There He laid himself as a foundation by which we may pass over—like a man laying concrete across a swamp ... However great the depth of sorrow or shame you or I may be in, it is not bottomless. He went lower still—so that we might pass over.[8]

And surely we can hope that such love will be fully revealed to all as they die and pass into the Presence.

For those around, both family and staff, comes the other phrase of Gethsemane: 'Watch with me'. When first uttered by Jesus it could not have meant 'take away', 'explain' or even understand'. Its simple but costly demand was plainly no more than just 'be there':

> Our most important foundation for St Christopher's is the hope that in watching we should learn not only how to free patients from pain and distress, how to understand them and never let them down, but also how to be silent, how to listen and how just to be there. As we learn this we will also learn that the real work is not ours at all.[9]

During the two decades since that was written the hospice movement, a movement facing death and long-term illness and bereavement, has come a long way, and has seen its basic principles interpreted in many settings and begin to move into the general hospital and community field. It has endeavoured to remove the fact and the fear of terminal distress by a combination of tough clinical science and personal attention to detail. It has seen the whole family as the unit of care and tried to help each group to discover their own strengths as they try to share as much of the truth of the situation as they can. Its workers have opened themselves to the angers and fears that make up the anguish of some of the dying and the bereaved. They have watched many people come along the journey from disbelief through gradual realisation to acceptance and offered what hospitality they could. In so doing they have often found themselves receivers rather than givers, gaining new strengths and insights from those they set out to help. To face death is to face life and to come to terms with one is to learn much about the other. In doing this the group have learnt also how much they need to share together their own experience of loss and change in this work. A hospice team needs to be some kind of a community. They have watched many people find that the God who Himself died is beside them and ready to give them courage and have seen Him more clearly for themselves:

> When He was born a man ... He put on the leaden shroud that's man's dying body. And on the Cross it bore Him down, sore heavy, dragging against the great nails, muffling God, blinding Him to the blindness of a man. But there, darkened within that shroud of mortal lead, beyond the furthest edge

of hope, God had courage to trust yet in hopeless, helpless things, in gentle mercy, holiness, love crucified.

And that courage, it was too rare and keen and quick a thing for sullen lead to prison, but instead it broke through, thinning lead, fining it to purest shining glass, to be a lamp for God to burn in. So men may have courage... Then they will see how bright God shines.[10]

The Christian answer to the mystery of suffering and death is not an explanation but a Presence. Alfred the Great translated Boethius as he cried out from the suffering of the Dark Ages. Our own cry today echoes his, and the answer is the same: 'Why has thou made me thus?' He will translate it, and after many days he will translate the answer, which is no answer in logic, but in excess of light.

> O Father, give the spirit power to climb
> To the fountain of all light, and be purified
> Break through the mists of earth, the weight of the clod,
> Shine forth in splendour, Thou that art calm weather,
> And quiet resting place for faithful souls.
> To see Thee is the end and the beginning,
> Thou carriest us, and Thou dost go before,
> Thou art the journey, and the journey's end.[11]

Notes

1. M. Wandor, 'Only half the story', in J. Garcia and S. Maitland (eds.), *Walking on the water: women talk about spirituality* (London: Virago, 1983), p. 103.
2. P. Teilhard de Chardin, *Le milieu divin. An essay on the interior life* (London: Collins, 1960), pp. 72–73.
3. H.Y. Vanderpool, 'The ethics of terminal care', *Journal of the American Medical Association*, vol. 239 (1978), pp. 850–52.
4. T.D. Walsh, 'Pain relief in cancer', *Medicine in practice*, vol. 1 (1983), pp. 684–89.
5. Anon., 'Death of a mind. A study in disintegration', *Lancet*, vol. 1, pp. 1012–15.
6. V. Frankl, *Man's search for meaning* (London: Hodder & Stoughton, 1962).

7. S. Du Boulay, 'Ramsey's diary', in *Cicely Saunders, the founder of the modern hospice movement* (London: Hodder & Stoughton, 1984), pp. 204–05.

8. B. Clements, quoted in the *The unity book of prayers* (London: Geoffrey Chapman, 1969), p. 103.

9. C. Saunders, 'Watch with Me', *Nursing Times*, vol. 61, no. 48 (1965), pp. 1615–17.

10. H.F.M. Prescott, *The man on a donkey* (New York: Macmillan, 1952), p. 1537.

11. H. Waddell, *Poetry in the dark ages* (London: Constable, 1948), p. 26.

A Personal Therapeutic Journey

I began training as a ward nurse in 1941 at St Thomas's Hospital. We had a limited pharmacopoeia, which gradually included sulphonamides but no other antibiotics, and few of the other drugs that we now take for granted. There were no diuretics, antihypertensive drugs, antiemetics or any psychotropic drugs beyond barbiturates and chloral. Linctus, mistura expectorans or mistura potassium iodide, and the evil-tasting potassium citrate were regularly prescribed, and much of what we offered would today be dismissed as 'custodial care'. We boiled up our 'porringers' for lotions, folded our dressings for autoclaving and reused our needles after a period in spirit. Operation days were a nightmare of vomiting patients.

Young patients dying of tuberculosis and septicaemia from war wounds begged us to save them somehow, but we had little to offer except devoted nursing. Osteomyelitis led to amputation and gastric ulcers to a milk diet. Penicillin appeared after D-day, when soldiers arrived saying that they could not face another blunt needle. We had morphine by injection but used it sparingly.

We worked a duty of 12 nights on, two nights off for three months, with split duties by day, and we had one day off a week from 5 PM the previous day. I was tired but deeply happy and satisfied. I have never lost touch with my set: the remaining members still meet regularly.

First published in the *British Medical Journal*, vol. 313 (21–28 December 1996), pp. 1599–1601, and appears here by kind permission of the BMJ Publishing Group.

Invalided out with back trouble, I returned to Oxford in 1944, completed a war degree, had a laminectomy, and became a lady almoner (now known as a medical social worker) back at St Thomas's.

Brompton cocktails

In March 1948 I began working as a volunteer nurse once or twice a week in one of the early homes for 'terminal care'. St Luke's Hospital had 48 beds for patients with advanced cancer. Here I met the regular administration of a modified 'Brompton cocktail' every four hours. The St Luke's version omitted the cannabis and, I think, the cocaine. They adjusted the morphine dose to the patient's need; if more than 60 mg was required the route was changed to injection. Hyoscine was used with morphine for terminal restlessness.

From 1951 to 1957 I was a medical student, yet again at St Thomas's. During that time there was a revolution in the drugs available for control of symptoms. The first phenothiazines, the antidepressants, the benzodiazepines, the synthetic steroids and the nonsteroidal anti-inflammatory drugs had all come into use by the time I arrived at St Joseph's Hospice in October 1958. A clinical research fellowship from the Department of Pharmacology at St Mary's Hospital Medical School under Professor Harold Stewart enabled me to begin work there to investigate terminal pain and its relief.

St Joseph's Irish Sisters of Charity had welcomed the local chest physician with the new antituberculosis drugs in the early 1950s and were ready for further innovations. The two visiting general practitioners were pleased to have help. They had already begun using chlorpromazine but they were not giving morphine orally or regularly, relying on injections as required and pethidine by mouth. Oral morphine together with alcohol and cocaine was introduced with cyclizine as the main antiemetic. The doses were nearly all as low as I had seen in St Luke's. The therapeutic advances and having the time to sit and listen to a patient's story, transformed the wards.

Gradually, we began to tackle the other symptoms. I tried

to set up a trial of nepenthe (an oral opioid) with or without aspirin but found the almost solo clinical care of patients in 45 beds made completion impossible. Instead, I was able to report to the Royal Society of Medicine in November 1962 on analysed records of 900 patients showing that 'tolerance and addiction are not problems to us, even with those who stay longest.'[1]

Greater confidence

We had by that time begun to use diamorphine. There were no controlled trials of this drug to be found, only some clinical reports that it had few side effects. We used it for 42 of our first 500 patients, in women with severe nausea and in a few patients with intolerable feelings of suffocation. By that time we believed that this was the drug of choice, but I realised two things. First, we were getting better and more confident in all that we were doing, secondly, that your own enthusiasms must be tested. The later work at St Christopher's Hospice by Twycross showed that there was no clinically observable difference between morphine and diamorphine given orally in our setting and with adjuvant treatment.[2]

During the seven years at St Joseph's between 1958 and 1965 we increased our pharmacopoeia, our patients' activities, their discharges and referrals back for radiotherapy. Gautier Smith came occasionally to perform nerve blocks. I wrote and lectured widely and produced a handout of the drugs in common use at St Joseph's and at St Christopher's Hospice, which opened in 1967. The handout has been updated, enlarged and reproduced widely. It has, of course, been joined by books and pamphlets from Twycross and others. We now have the *Oxford textbook of palliative medicine*. The fundamentals of therapeutics I believe remain as I wrote in 1963:

> We believe that there are a few cardinal rules in the treatment of intractable pain at this stage. First, we have to make as careful an assessment as possible of the symptoms that trouble the patient. This is not in order to make a diagnosis and give specific treatment, because that has already been

done, but in order to treat pain and all the other things that can add up to a general state of misery as a disease in itself.[3]

It soon became clear that each death was as individual as the life that preceded it and that the whole experience of that life was reflected in a patient's dying. This led to the concept of 'total pain', which was presented as a complex of physical, emotional, social and spiritual elements. The whole experience for a patient includes anxiety, depression and fear; concern for the family who will become bereaved; and often a need to find some meaning in the situation, some deeper reality in which to trust. This became the major emphasis of much lecturing and writing on subjects such as the nature and management of terminal pain and the family as the unit of care.[4]

Importance of active total care

It was recognised that support was needed both before and after a patient's death, particularly in home care, when the family are the central carers. The World Health Organisation has published the following definition:

> Palliative care is the active total care of patients whose disease is not responsive to curative treatment. Control of pain, of other symptoms and of psychological, social and spiritual problems is paramount. The goal of palliative care is achievement of the best possible quality of life for patients and their families.[5]

The basic and clinical researchers, together with many clinicians—doctors, nurses and many in auxiliary services—have enlarged our detailed knowledge of physical pain since that was written. The emphasis on regular giving has been accepted widely and also features as an essential element in relieving the pain of cancer. It is one of the cardinal principles of the WHO booklet *Cancer pain relief*, available in many languages and now in a second edition.[6] Over 33 years later, these basic principles have not changed, although symptomatic treatment is far more complex and specialists in palliative care have to keep abreast of developments in all relevant disciplines.

Many therapeutic discoveries of recent years have been relevant to palliative care. For example, the pharmacological management of terminal bowel obstruction has been improved with the use of octreotide. Hypercalcaemia is now identified and treated with bisphosphonates. In the drive to question received wisdom, investigations continue into the best and appropriate ways of treating dyspnoea and the problems arising from dehydration (not always symptomatic). Neuropathic pain is better managed but still needs further work. Looking ahead, I sometimes wonder that if we are not careful we may see a postantibiotic era. Whatever happens, it will still matter that we go on listening and that we continue our questioning. Above all, my experience emphasises that the practice of medicine includes more than specific treatments.

We were the hosts

The advances in pharmacology and the new technologies are not the whole story. At our preliminary training school we were taught that we were host to our patients and their visiting families. It was also taken for granted that we would join in ward prayers morning and evening and carry out 'last offices' with reverence and respect. Life has changed greatly in over 55 years, but people's needs, though expressed differently, remain beyond the strictly physical. Palliative care physicians are not to be merely 'symptomologists', as Kearney has expressed it.[7]

Now that palliative care is spreading worldwide it has still, as in the WHO definition, kept a concern for the spiritual needs of its patients and their families. The whole approach has been based on the understanding that a person is an indivisible entity, a physical and a spiritual being. 'The only proper response to a person is respect; a way of seeing and listening to each one in the whole context of their culture and relationships, thereby giving each his or her intrinsic value'.[8] The search for meaning, for something in which to trust, may be expressed in many ways, direct and indirect, in metaphor or silence, in gesture or symbol or, perhaps most all, in art and the unexpected potential for creativity at the end of life.

Those who work in palliative care may have to realise that they, too, are being challenged to face this dimension for themselves. Many, both helper and patient, live in a secularised society and have no religious language. Some will, of course, still be in touch with their religious roots and find a familiar practice, liturgy, or sacrament to help their need. Others, however, will not. For them, insensitive suggestions by well-meaning practitioners will be unwelcome. However, if we can come not only in our professional capacity but in our common, vulnerable humanity there may be no need of words on our part, only of concerned listening. For those who do not wish to share their deepest needs, the way care is given can reach the most hidden places. Feelings of fear and guilt may seem inconsolable, but many of us have sensed that an inner journey has taken place and that a person nearing the end of life has found peace. Important relationships may be developed or reconciled at this time and a new sense of self worth develop. A recent study shows how this may happen in late modern social conditions.[9]

My personal therapeutic journey has witnessed an extraordinary growth in drug treatments for pain and other symptoms. The challenge of educating others on their use remains. However, there has always been a human as well as a professional basis that is fundamental to the work that we do. Everyone meeting these patients and their families is challenged to have some awareness of this dimension. Professionals' own search for meaning can create a climate, as we tried often helplessly to do all those years ago, in which patients and families can reach out in trust towards what they see as true and find courage and acceptance of what is happening to them.

Notes

1. C. Saunders, 'The treatment of intractable pain in terminal cancer', *Proceedings of the Royal Society of Medicine*, vol. 56 (1963), pp. 195–97.

2. R. Twycross, 'Choice of strong analgesic in terminal cancer care: morphine or diamorphine?', *Pain*, vol. 3 (1977), pp. 93–104.

3. C. Saunders, 'The challenge of terminal care', in T. Symington and R.L. Carter (eds.), *Scientific foundations of oncology* (London: Heinemann Medical Books, 1976), pp. 673–79.

4. C. Saunders, 'The care of the dying patient and his family', *Contact*, vol. 38 (1972), pp. 12–18.

5. World Health Organisation, *Cancer pain relief* (Geneva: WHO, 1996).

6. World Health Organisation Expert Committee, *Report. Cancer pain relief and palliative care* (Geneva: WHO, 1990), p. 11.

7. M. Kearney, 'Palliative medicine—just another specialty?', *Palliative Medicine*, vol. 6 (1992), pp. 39–46.

8. M. Mayne, personal communication (1992).

9. C. Seale, 'Heroic death', *Sociology*, vol. 29 (1995), pp. 597–613.

Consider Him

On my desk I have a framed photograph of a crucifix from the rebuilt cathedral of Warsaw, razed to the ground at the end of the Resistance. The crucifix was burned, bombed and shot at and the twisted metal figure hangs by one arm from the charred cross. It continually says to me, 'This is what Warsaw did to God' and, 'This is what God endlessly shares with us.' It echoes Dietrich Bonhoeffer, writing from prison 'only a suffering God can help'.[1]

It also pictures the God of daily hospice work. As our chaplain says, 'There may be a Good Friday here, but this is also an Easter place.' I personally do not see much of the patients and families at St Christopher's now, but what I do see still lifts my heart (last week it was a hug from the grateful wife of a patient). I was waiting recently in our reception area when a man called in to light a candle in our chapel. As he thanked me for the care of the hospice, he added, 'my wife was very happy here.' A place where the sacraments of the cup of cold water and the feet washing go on continually (often by people whose service is simply to care without any acknowledged spiritual commitment) gives such a welcome to all.

My journey to that wait in reception began as I searched for God during my wartime nursing. The work of C.S. Lewis, Dorothy Sayers's *The man born to be king*[2] and Helen Waddell's

Given as a lecture in Westminster Cathedral Hall in June 2003 as part of a series arranged by Christian Life Community on 'The spiritual exercises of St Ignatius in the varieties of human experience'.

Peter Abelard,[3] together with the faith of members of my training set, led eventually in 1945 to a moment of coming to God 'without one plea'. I was told in my heart just to accept. I believed God said 'I've done it all' and I felt as I turned round—or was turned?—that the wind that had been so long in my face was now at my back.

The next three years were spent in training and hospital social work, as I had been invalided out from nursing. Joining All Souls and an evangelical group, I was steeped in Bible study (for which I remain deeply grateful). I did not, however, know what else was expected of me until July 1947, when I met David Tasma, a Jew from Warsaw who had advanced cancer. After his discharge from hospital, I followed him up in Outpatients as I knew that, as a solitary man in digs, he was bound to run into trouble. In January 1948 he was admitted to another hospital and during the next two months I was his constant and virtually only visitor. We talked around his life of only 40 years and his lost faith, together with his feeling that he had done nothing for which the world would remember him. We discussed a Home I might found to meet the needs of symptom control and individual recognition at the end of life. He talked of his legacy— he left me £500 saying, 'I will be a window in your Home.' On another evening he suddenly said, 'Can't you say something to comfort me?' Respecting his Jewishness, I repeated Psalm 23 and then the Venite and 'I will lift up mine eyes'. Although much choir singing had enabled me to remember these by heart, I then suggested reading from a book in my bag of Psalms and the New Testament. 'No,' he said, 'I only want what is in your mind and in your heart.' I learned the De Profundis that night for him and he later said to his ward sister, 'I have made my peace with the God of my fathers.' He died a few days later. His employer and I were the only mourners as we said Psalm 91 for him at his funeral.

Two days later I went to an All Souls prayer meeting. We began to sing 'How sweet the name of Jesus sounds' and I said to myself, 'But it didn't to him' and I felt myself as it were, tapped on the shoulder, and told, 'He knows me now far better than you do.' That message of assurance for all who would pass into Paradise, however unbelieving, has remained with me ever since. David had found his way in the freedom of the spirit. This with the challenge of openness from the symbol of the window, the match of all the diligence of the mind together with the vulnerability of the heart, these were the founding principles of hospice and palliative care and, I believe, still stand today. David's window is part of the main reception at St Christopher's Hospice and is a wonderful heritage that sends a message around the world.

It took me 19 years to build the Home around the window. I went through medical training and much research and exploration. Working in an early Protestant home for end of life care as a volunteer evening nurse, I was assured that indeed this was my calling. I also saw how the nurses had instituted the regular giving of oral morphine with far better pain relief than I had ever seen before. After three years I was impelled into medicine by the surgeon I was working for 'because there's so much more to be learned about pain and you'll only be frustrated if you don't do it properly—and they won't listen to you'.[4]

Arriving at St Joseph's Hospice in October 1958, I found few patient records and drugs being given on demand, patients (as elsewhere) having to earn their morphine by experiencing pain first. Marvellously loving care was being given by the Irish Sisters of Charity who welcomed me, as a Protestant, before Vatican II. The years spent there in detailed care and research, where I gradually introduced the regular giving of medication that I had witnessed previously, are the first scientific foundations of care for dying people. During the war, we had so often nothing to offer but ourselves, now we had new resources to add to our compassion.

I was helped through my student years by my fellows (all much younger) but also by Mrs G, a patient. Barbara Galton was a young, blind and increasingly paralysed patient who was in branches of St Thomas' Hospital for the seven years I knew her. Her story is one of triumph and a precious friendship full of laughter. She came to believe through her illness. She once said to a medical student, 'Some people can read their Bibles and get their help there, some people go to Church and get their help there—but He deals with me differently, He sends me people.' Many of these were members of an extremely open and relaxed Christian Union and her influence spread widely. Among other gifts, she gave St Christopher's its name. 'Hospice? A stopping place for travellers? Well, you'll have to call it St Christopher's, won't you.' Thousands, even millions, around the world have been helped on their personal journey since then.

On 24 June 1959 my daily Bible reading said, 'Commit thy way unto the Lord and He shall bring it to pass.' Once again God tapped me on the shoulder—'Now you must get on with it.' After a personal retreat, I wrote the first Scheme of the need and the project and, with the help of a gathering of personal friends, we were underway.

In 1960 I met Olive Wyon, our ecumenical theologian and Bishop Evered Lunt of Stepney, our spiritual director. We looked at how an open Christian Foundation should be expressed and how to establish a community that would have some of the underpinning strength I had seen at St Joseph's Hospice. Two or three of the nuns there, with no trace of jealousy, became as excited as we were as the interest and funds began to come in. As for a community, after much heart-searching it was laid aside—'we will know when we get there'—and we have gone on learning together. My letters and daily prayer diary of these years reveal the intensity of the search and the many setbacks.

We began meeting as a steering committee in 1960 and, two years later, drew together a larger group to meet with the Bishop and Dr Wyon and to get to know each other as we discussed the foundations of the future hospice. We began before we had the land. A group of current staff inherits the discussion and debate begun by that group and meets regularly to talk about the spiritual needs of patients today. This group is I have to say, as we share our experiences, often merry and exhilarating. The hospice's original Aim and Basis of 1965 refers to the development as 'group work, open to further light and expansion, as the Holy Spirit may lead'. A revised and shortened draft in 1992 added, 'The wider spiritual dimension at St Christopher's has been built up from the creativity and growth of many of its patients and witnesses to the discovery of their own strengths by countless families; it has also developed through the experience of the staff, a community of the unlike.' It adds that 'it was established and has grown as a Christian Foundation, not simply in terms of its care but from a belief that the God revealed in Christ shared and shares in the darkness of suffering and dying and has transformed the reality of death'. Many now working here would not subscribe to the latter statement but the foundations are there, even if hidden. The Chapel is below the four wards and is frequently visited by family members and friends, who light candles, take cards and leave requests for prayer. The current chaplaincy team responds to countless referrals and demands and over and over again people remark on the hospice as being a place of spiritual peace. It is also a place of laughter, with much of the humour coming from the patients themselves.

God had an unexpected way of giving authenticity to this search. In February 1960 I admitted to St Joseph's an ex-Eighth Army Polish refugee, Antoni Michniewicz, aged 60, suffering from sarcoma. For five months he was a challenging, courteous patient. I was making tape recordings of patients talking of their pain and their feelings as part of my research. The only one I have of him is of him laughing about English cooking. But in July when his daughter (he was a widower) passed her exams, she said something about his feelings for me that suddenly unmade my world. During the next few weeks we lived a lifetime, all in a six-bed patient bay. What came next is recorded both in my prayer diary and an evening record of each day until he died three-and-a-half weeks later.

His journey went from 'I do not *want* to die, I do not *want* to die' to 'I only want what is right'. I travelled that journey with him, a journey of physical diminishment and growing love. Olive Wyon had set me to read Teilhard de Chardin's *Le milieu divin*[5] early in 1960. His writing of life's passivities was underlined in our intense, private yet public experience. It is not an easy story to tell or for you to understand. Reading my diary I see again the humiliations of Antoni's dependence and my rigorous discipline (curtains only pulled as for any other patient). I wrote of some precious hours from 5 to 6 PM when we could talk, knowing that the silence for which we longed would have been impossible. We both tried to talk of this to the wonderfully kind ward sister, but she didn't realise what we were experiencing and just said, 'Nothing can come between Mr M and God.' One day, on looking at the crucifix on the wall opposite, he suddenly said, 'I can see my Saviour' and I replied, 'He is my Saviour too, so wherever we are we will be together. When you are gone He will still be here and it will be alright.' I went to the hospice every day, but could never telephone first to see if he was still there. 'I am waiting till you come, but I can give you nothing, nothing but sorrow,' he said. Ten days before he died I stopped asking God for a little more time and took my hands off. God then gave us quiet hearts and a timeless moment when Antoni finally believed he was the giver too. I was there all his last day, although not at the moment he died. It was the Feast of the Assumption, a wonderful day for a devout Polish Catholic to die. I lifted him up once to see the crucifix—the only time I had held him. Just before he finally lost consciousness he gave me what I described that evening in my diary as a 'really heavenly smile. And as I think of it I am not certain of all that was in it. Not sorrow at all, it looked so happy and there was certainly a gleam of amusement and somehow strong. And then that look of pure love I have had so often.' He died with his daughter and ward sister beside him an hour later (they had not been able to be there throughout the day).

Next day I went in as usual but I remember standing at the door and seeing another patient in his bed and thinking 'I can't go in, it hurts too much.' Then I looked at the crucifix and let it hold me. But I found I couldn't really think and stayed for the next five days with a wonderfully understanding widowed friend who knew of my need. Much of what I read afterwards on my journey are gathered together in a little anthology *Beyond the horizon* which also includes many poems written by St Christopher's patients. It is a search for meaning in suffering.[6]

The prayer diary records the next bleak two-and-a-half years of a walk through a cold and dark tunnel and endless work at St Joseph's and planning for St Christopher's. Mrs G died five months later and my father six months after that. I see now that I got my bereavements muddled up but my most vivid memories are of learning hymns, mystical poems and Psalms by heart and of using a rosary for the Orthodox Jesus Prayer to steady my thoughts. Above all I found a kind of a ladder out of the dark hole of grief. The two uprights were 'Oh my love how happy you are' and 'O God I am so grateful', and each time I reached this I came back to find that there was another rung to climb on to.

After all these years, countless visits to St Julian's (now St Cuthmans) in Sussex for quiet reading and peaceful bird watching, much music and many exciting trips to visit new pioneers of hospice worldwide, as well as a late but deeply happy marriage to yet another Pole, I still sometimes need that ladder to help with an abiding sense of loss. However, I have no regrets about a meeting that could have happened in no other time or place and am certain that bereavement can bring gifts of creative energy. We see this so often in the parents who have lost a child and who then dedicate their lives to charities in that child's name.

One patient in St Joseph's summed it up for me when she showed me a poem about suffering with the words, 'Tell me about this doctor, I know you know.' The patients of those next years were, one by one, founders of the modern hospice movement.[7]

Alongside David, Antoni and Mrs G, I place another patient, Louie, as a key teacher. In bed all her life with fragile bones, she reached St Joseph's just before I did and she and two companions in her bay joined in every detail of the planning of St Christopher's. Like me she was an Anglican, happily welcomed to that Catholic milieu. Once in one of our many conversations, I found myself saying 'What's the first thing you will say to Him, Louie?' Without any hesitation she said simply 'I know You.' I believe that she speaks for all who will wake to His light and that the desperate, wounded unbelievers will also say in wonder, 'I know You, You were there.' We cannot go beyond the reach of His self-giving love. People may say, 'But what about free will, a free rejection?' and I can only say that I believe the true vision will lead to a final turning towards Him. When we fall in love we feel we cannot help it and yet looking back, it is a moment of true freedom. So, I believe, it is with God.

One of my pillars of wisdom is Mother Julian's book *Revelations of divine love*.[8] I have read and re-read it in every new translation I could find, even the original with a crib. She saw no wrath in God, but that He sees us with pity, not with blame. Julian questioned with much heartache how all shall be well as God told her, and He promised a Great Deed at the end. While keeping to the teachings of Holy Church, she yet edges towards a hopeful universal vision as she talks of all who will be saved.

As Bishop John Austin Baker wrote in his formative book *The faith of a Christian*:

> The traditional picture of judgement is shot through with anomalies and contradictions—it asks us to believe that God's attitude towards us changes radically the moment we die. While we are in this life, forgiveness and reconciliation are available whenever we are truly sorry and forgive others. But it would seem that as soon as we die, love and mercy are out. From then on unrepented sin committed in this life excludes us forever from the joy of life in the family of God.[9]

In *The foolishness of God* he also writes 'the crucified Jesus is the only accurate picture of God the world has ever seen, and the hands that hold us in existence are pierced with unimaginable nails.'[10] Such desperately vulnerable love can surely never finally be defeated.

The simple statement to Antoni, 'I love you because you are you', became translated, during the years of listening to countless patients, to the watchwords, 'You matter because you are you and you matter to the end of your life. We will do all we can not only to help you die peacefully, but also to live until you die.'

This welcome has been founded on the research begun at St Joseph's, where I summarised 1,100 patient notes on punch cards (this was before computers). I was able to show that the textbook teaching that morphine by mouth had little effect, that doses inevitably escalated as tolerance and drug dependence developed and that patients therefore had inevitably to wait until the very end, was completely wrong. We showed then, and continue to demonstrate, that patients with advanced cancer can be relieved of pain and able to live as themselves in their homes, in day centres, as well as inpatients. There are the complexities of total pain that I first described in 1964.[11] These are the physical, emotional/mental, social/family and spiritual aspects that combine to give the complex pain so many suffer. Staff pain was added some years later. We are continually learning but all suffering cannot be wished or medicated away. There is still 'much to be learned about pain' but it can be transmuted into the treasures of darkness. One never becomes used to the pain in peoples' eyes and I am sure that parting is the worst pain of all and that in many ways, dying is easier to face than bereavement.

Spiritual pain is a challenging reality. Viktor Frankl's book *Man's search for meaning* was written about experiences in the death camp he survived. His assurance that the last freedom is to choose one's attitude in any given set of circumstances, to choose one's own way,[12] is also recognised and met in hospice care. A report from a qualitative study of the existential experience reached me as I began work on this talk. It confirms Viktor Frankl's assertion, but goes on to say that meaning is not an end in itself, but a catalyst for an enhanced sense of connectedness and on into the present moment when healing occurs. I have often said that we see the healing of wholeness and of many little resurrections. I recall the man with motor neurone disease who looked at another patient who was further along that path of diminishment and commented, 'If I ever get like that chap I'll do something to myself.' When he did get to that point, he said simply, 'I can't see round the next bend but I know it will be alright.' While many people express a deep sense of accountability to the chaplain, few patients today use overtly religious language. Like this patient, they employ metaphors to express their personal spiritual journey (he had called his a 'coming together illness'), and we often see reconciliation and peace come without any words.

Coming together—with all those remembered in Paradise (who are all so much part of my often wandering daily prayers) but above all, with 'the creative suffering of God'. As the Baptist theologian Paul Fiddes has presented it in his powerful book of that title, 'Death becomes a place where we trust God to preserve our relationship with Him and others—the sign of the resurrection of Jesus affirms that God does something new for His creation in face of the finality of death.'[13] Words are my way into prayer. My Psalter is marked with many names and dates but none are remembered so vividly as a few weeks after Antoni died when Psalm 132 said to me, 'We will go into his tabernacle and fall low on our knees before his footstool.' Each month I reach it with thanks.

There are no easy answers—there are many times when only a crucifix can hold you, when the only prayer is 'Jesus— Saviour' and 'Thou knowest', when the only response is not words but a presence. Hospice and palliative care today is carried out by many people who find religious answers do not speak to them. Nevertheless they give much spiritual help. When I asked our chaplain what was the real foundation for his work, he said simply 'brokenness'. He meant having nothing to say but the giving of a listening presence. Surely 'Watch with me' could not have meant to take away or explain or even understand—it simply meant 'be there'. Alongside this, the way care is given can reach the most hidden places. You do not have to be brokenhearted as I was and for which I am so grateful, but you do have to face all the little deaths of living in this free and very dangerous world. You may feel helpless and only able to share the pain—but that is the connectedness in which the helpless Christ comes incognito to meet those dying members of his family. As Father Congreve wrote:

> Christ by his sacrifice for us, by the self-emptying of the Incarnation, acquired a new power of stealing into wounded and sorrowful hearts in their extremest dejection and dryness. He comes by His saving death to dying people ... The mystery of Christ's love in death can steal into that

silence, and fill that supreme emptiness ... In the hour of death and the day of judgement, Good Lord, deliver us.[14]

Many years ago I took some photographs of a patient at a party. He wanted to pay, I wanted to give them to him. We both wanted to give, not to receive. I put my hand out next to his, palm upright and said, 'I suppose that is what life is about, learning to receive.' He put both his hands out next to mine. 'That's what life is about, four hands held out together.' As we hold out our hands together, it is to the crucified but risen Christ.

Among the many who pray for us daily are the nuns of the contemplative Anglican convent at Tymawr, Monmouth. From them comes the poem 'Fresh Springs' from my anthology with which I end:

> That perfect balance
> Between agony and joy
> Given
> Through His Cross and Resurrection.
> The loving touch
> Of His hands
> Heals
> Our wounded hearts and spirits
> Making them whole.
> His loving patience
> With us,
> His compassion for us
> Blesses us
> With fresh springs of love:
> Unutterable joy.[15]

Notes

1. D. Bonhoffer, *Letters and papers from prison* (London: Fontana Books, 1959), p. 122.
2. D.L. Sayers, *The man born to be king* (London: Victor Gollancz, 1943).
3. H. Waddell, *Peter Abelard* (London: Constable, 1933).
4. N.R. Barrett, personal communication (1951).
5. P. Teilhard de Chardin, *Le milieu divin. An essay on the interior life* (London: Collins, 1960).

6. C. Saunders, *Beyond the horizon* (London: Darton, Longman & Todd, 1990).

7. D. Clark, 'Originating a Movement: Cicely Saunders and the development of St Christopher's Hospice 1957–67', *Mortality*, vol. 3, no. 1 (1998), pp. 43–63.

8. Julian of Norwich, *Revelations of Divine Love* (New York: Doubleday, 1997, trans. J. Skinner).

9. J.A. Baker, *The faith of a Christian* (London: Darton, Longman & Todd, 1996), p. 125.

10. J.A. Baker, *The foolishness of God* (London: Darton, Longman & Todd, 1970), p. 406.

11. C. Saunders, 'The symptomatic treatment of incurable malignant disease', *Prescribers Journal*, vol. 4 (1964), pp. 68–73.

12. V.E. Frankl, *Man's search for meaning* (London: Hodder & Stoughton, 1962), p. 66.

13. P.S. Fiddes, *The creative suffering of God* (Oxford, Clarendon Press, 1988, p. 267).

14. Fr. Congreve, quoted in O. Wyon, *Consider Him: three meditations on the Passion Story* (London: SCM Press, 1956), quoted in Saunders, *Beyond the horizon*, p. 45.

15. Sr Gillian Mary S.S.C. (Society of the Sacred Cross), 'Fresh Springs', in Saunders, *Beyond the horizon*, p. 79.

Mortal Press

Innovative Writing on End-of-Life Issues

Human mortality is a rare constant in a changing world. Yet how we die is a matter of growing social, medical and moral complexity and creates one of the major challenges of our times. Mortal Press promotes the understanding of death, dying and bereavement; seeks to improve care at the end of life; fosters interdisciplinary perspectives; and encourages the most innovative writers, editors and researchers in the field.

Mortal Press focuses on the following areas:

- Historical and cultural studies of hospice, palliative care and related end of life issues

- Studies of current issues in the development of palliative care both nationally and internationally, focusing on service development, policy factors and reimbursement issues

- Empirical and theoretical contributions on mortality and end of life issues from anthropology, sociology, social psychology, ethics, religious studies and the clinical disciplines

Founded in 2003 by the sociologist Professor David Clark, Mortal Press is located within the International Observatory on End of Life Care at Lancaster University. Proceeds from the sale of Mortal Press publications are used to support the work of the Observatory which operates on a non-profit basis.

For full details of current and forthcoming titles, and how to purchase Mortal Press books, please see www.mortalpress.com or write to us at:

MORTAL PRESS
PO Box 625
Sheffield S1 3GY
United Kingdom

info@mortalpress.com